# Table of Contents

## Kegel Exercises

Kegel exercises are designed to strengthen the pelvic floor muscles. These muscles support the bladder and bowel openings in both men and women. Strengthening the muscles of the pelvic floor can aid in preventing leakage of urine or feces with coughing, sneezing, lifting, and other stressful movements. Other benefits of kegels include enhanced sexual function, conditioned muscles to make childbirth easier, decrease and/or prevent prolapse of pelvic organs, and improve the ability to pass stool.

## Kegel or Pelvic Floor Muscle Exercises for Men

Prostate cancer surgery or radiation treatment can weaken the muscles around your bladder. When this happens, you may start to have problems with urinary incontinence or a lack of bladder control. These are characterized by the leaking or passing of urine on accident.

Pelvic floor muscles can be made weaker by:

• Surgery for bladder or bowel problems

• Constipation

• Being overweight

• Heavy lifting

• Long-term coughing (such as smoker's cough, bronchitis, or asthma)

• Being unfit

Kegels, or pelvic floor muscle exercises, can help strengthen the muscles to regain your control or prepare for pelvic surgery.

## What are the pelvic floor muscles?

The pelvic floor is made up of layers of muscle and other tissue that stretch like a hammock from the tailbone, forward to the pubic bone.

A man's pelvic floor muscles support his bladder and bowel (colon) while allowing the urine tube (urethra) and rectum to pass through. Your pelvic floor muscles help you to control your bladder, bowel, and sexual function. In order to maintain control after surgery or radiation treatment, it is vital to keep your pelvic floor muscles strong.

## How do I find the right muscles?

To find the right muscles, try the following:

• The next time you urinate, try to start and stop your urine stream. This will help you find the correct muscles.

• Do not tighten your buttocks or thigh muscles when doing these exercises.

• Relax your stomach muscles as much as possible.

• When you are standing and squeeze your pelvic floor muscles, you should see your penis move slightly.

## Who should do Kegel exercises?

• Women and men with urinary and /or bowel incontinence

• Women and men who have demonstrated weakening of the pelvic floor

• Pregnant women or women who have previously had children

• Middle aged and older women

## What you need to know about Kegels

The success of Kegel exercises depends on the use of proper technique as well as compliance to a regular exercise program. When doing the exercises, it is important to identify the correct muscles of the pelvic floor. At first, most people contract the abdominal or thigh muscles while neglecting the pelvic floor muscles. This may actually worsen pelvic floor tone and incontinence.

Kegels may be done as a part of biofeedback, when some patients require assistance. Biofeedback consists of placing a sensor on the abdomen and around the anal area, which measure the contraction of the pelvic floor muscles. Occasionally, an electrode may be placed in the vagina in women, or in the rectum in men.

## Steps to an effective Kegel

• Learn to tighten the muscles around the vaginal/anal area

• Contract the vaginal and rectal muscles. Note that when you perform steps 1 and 2 correctly, you should also feel the muscles around the anus tighten slightly. This is normal, but do not consciously try to tighten those muscles.

• In a quiet, relaxed setting with no distractions, practice your Kegels and determine how long you can hold your contraction and how many you can do before becoming fatigued. Do not do more than 5-10 reps at time with a 3-5 second hold.

## Basic Kegel Exercises
Detailed instructions for doing Kegel exercises

### Step 1: The urethra—The Functional Stop Test

After partially emptying your bladder, stop your urine flow in a slow controlled manner, paying attention to how it feels.

NOTE: Stopping and starting the urine repeatedly as an exercise can be harmful and should not be done. Holding your urine can contribute to bladder infection, causing damage to normal urinary reflexes. The Functional Stop Test is useful for assessing what it feels like to gradually stop urine flow, and should not be done more than once per urination.

### Step 2: The vagina and rectum as your window to the pelvic floor For this step, you will internally assess the ability to squeeze and elevate the muscles around the opening of the vagina or rectum, while lying on your back. This is

accomplished by inserting one finger into the vaginal or rectal opening while you try to lift and squeeze with the muscles. Pay attention to how this feels.

NOTE: For those who may be unable to check internally, you can place the pad of one finger on the perineal body (the area between the vagina and the anus) and assess for lift in this manner. The internal assessment is preferable, however, because it gives you a better sense of what you are capable of doing with your pelvic floor and provides a way to assess the strength and control you gain as you progress with your Kegels.

Step 3: Putting it all together

Begin practicing while lying on your back with your knees bent, or lying back with pillows under your head and shoulders. When your knees are bent you should have pillows under them so that the muscles around the hips and buttocks can relax. In this position, you can practice the actual

Kegel, which involves lifting and tightening the pelvic floor all at one time.

This will be a combination of what you felt when you gradually stopped urine flow, with the feeling squeezing and elevating the muscles around the vaginal or rectal area.

Step 4:

1. Sit or lie down with the muscles of your thighs and buttocks relaxed. It may be helpful to use a hand mirror to watch your pelvic floor muscles.

2. Squeeze the pelvic floor muscles and hold for a count of five (5), then relax for a count of five (5).

3. Do not squeeze your buttocks or bear down

4. You should feel a distinct "squeeze and lift" if done correctly.

5. Work up to doing the exercises five (5) times a day in sets of 10 (50 total per day).

Note: At first, you may not be able to hold the squeeze for 1 to 2 seconds, but you should aim for 5 as your muscles get stronger.

Step 5:

This exercise works on the ability of the muscles to "hold" over a length of time, building a strong dam to hold back urine.

Slowly lift and draw in the pelvic floor muscles and hold to a count of . Then, release.

Rest for seconds in between each contraction. Rest is just as important as the exercise, so never skip this step.

Once you have rested, contract your muscles again.

Do this exercise in the position.

Repeat times.

Do this times per day.

Step 6:

The second exercise is a quick contraction. The muscles are quickly tightened, lifted up, and let go, working the muscles that quickly shut off the flow of urine (like a faucet) to help prevent accidents. This exercise helps improve the ability of your muscles to respond quickly when you sneeze, cough, or make sudden changes in your position.

Squeeze your muscles quickly and strongly for just a second or two.

Release the contraction for just the moment, and contract again.

Your goal is to do repetitions of this exercise times a day.

Begin with as many as you can, and build up to this goal.

Do this exercise in the position.

Make sure to relax the pelvic floor between each repetition.

Step 7:

The "Knack" For Individuals with Stress Incontinence

Squeeze your pelvic floor by doing a quick contraction (as noted above)during activities such as coughing, laughing or sneezing. This decreases the chance you will leak.

Practice this throughout the day, as needed.

## Tips For Success

With practice and dedication, you can take control of your urinating habits and strengthen your pelvic floor muscles. Here are some helpful tips.

• Do kegel exercises anytime, anywhere! Try to incorporate them into your daily routine.

• Drink up – Your body needs fluids, so be sure to drink enough to stay well hydrated.

But, don't drink too much at night.

Sip on fluids during the day instead of gulping quickly to reduce urinary frequency and urgency.

Stop fluids two hours before bedtime to decrease getting up at night.

• Reduce fluids that can irritate the bladder, such as coffee, soda, tea, alcohol and sugar substitutes, and limit citrus drinks.

• Elevate your legs in the evening. This helps your kidneys to produce more urine so you can eliminate more before bedtime.

• Do not urinate "just-in-case."

• Never strain to urinate or strain during a bowel movement.

• Take your time when you're in the bathroom. After you've finished urinating, relax a bit, and then urinate again. This practice, called double voiding, really helps empty the bladder.

• Squeeze before you sneeze! Maintain a constant contraction throughout any activity that would cause a leak (cough, sneeze, laugh, lifting, positional changes). Make this a lifetime habit.

• Increase fiber intake to 20-30 grams a day. Increasing fiber can help prevent constipation. Being constipated presses on the bladder and may cause urinary urgency. Increasing fiber intake is not recommended for everyone; discuss your fiber needs with your medical provider.

• Quit smoking. Cigarette smoking irritates the bladder and is associated with bladder cancer. In addition, coughing associated with smoking may lead to increased incontinent episodes.

• Women can try wearing a tampon to help control leaks when jogging, running, dancing, or engaging in other energetic activities. The tampon puts a bit of pressure on your urethra, helping to prevent leakage.

• Remember to fill out your voiding diary (placed in the front pocket of your packet at your appointment) to monitor improvements.

• If you are overweight (as diagnosed by your medical provider), work with your provider, nutritionist or dietician, and develop a weight-loss plan to reach a healthier weight.

Weight loss of 5-10% has been shown to help decrease urinary incontinence symptoms by decreasing the pressure from the abdomen onto the bladder. Being overweight can also lead to diabetes, which can lead to urinary incontinence.

# ADVANCED KEGEL TECHNIQUES

## Incorporating Resistance And Weight Training Into Your Kegel Routine

Incorporating resistance and weight training into your Kegel routine can take your pelvic floor strength to the next level. Just like with any other muscle in the body, adding resistance can challenge and strengthen the pelvic floor muscles even more than simple contractions alone. One effective way to add resistance to Kegel exercises is by using Kegel balls or vaginal weights. These are small, weighted devices that can be inserted into the vagina and held in place by the pelvic floor muscles. By contracting around the weight, the muscles are forced to work harder than they would during a simple Kegel contraction. When starting with Kegel balls or weights, it's important to choose a size and weight that is appropriate for your current level of pelvic floor strength. If the weight is too heavy, it can actually cause more harm than good by putting too much pressure on the muscles. It's recommended to start with a lighter weight and gradually work your way up as your strength improves. To use Kegel balls or weights, begin by inserting them into the vagina and holding them in place with your pelvic floor muscles. You can then perform regular Kegel contractions, focusing on squeezing the muscles around the weight. As you get stronger, you can increase the number of repetitions or hold the weight in place for longer periods of time. Another way to add resistance to Kegel exercises is by using a resistance band. This can be particularly effective for men who are looking to strengthen their pelvic floor muscles. To use a resistance band for Kegels, wrap the band around the base of the penis and anchor it to a stable surface, such as a table or chair leg. You can then perform Kegel contractions against the resistance of the band, similar to how you would perform a bicep curl with a resistance band. When incorporating resistance or weight training into your Kegel routine, it's important to remember that proper form is key. Just like with any other exercise, using incorrect form can lead to injury or strain. Make sure to fully relax your pelvic floor muscles between contractions and avoid holding your breath or tensing other muscles during the exercise. It's also important to listen to your body and avoid pushing yourself too hard. If you experience pain or discomfort during the exercise, stop immediately and consult with a healthcare provider or pelvic floor physical therapist. Incorporating resistance and weight training into your Kegel routine can be a highly effective way to increase pelvic floor strength and improve sexual health and overall wellness. By gradually increasing the intensity of your Kegel exercises, you can achieve stronger, healthier pelvic floor muscles and enjoy the benefits of improved bladder control, better sexual function, and increased confidence.

# USING BIOFEEDBACK DEVICES TO TRACK YOUR PROGRESS

Biofeedback is a technique that involves monitoring and providing feedback on biological processes that are typically involuntary or unconscious, such as heart rate, blood pressure, and muscle tension. Biofeedback devices can be useful tools for tracking your progress with Kegel exercises, as they provide real-time information on the activity of your pelvic floor muscles. There are several types of biofeedback devices available for use with Kegel exercises, including vaginal sensors, anal sensors, and surface electromyography (EMG) sensors. These devices typically work by measuring the electrical activity of your pelvic floor muscles, which is then displayed on a screen or monitor. One advantage of using biofeedback devices is that they can help you to ensure that you are performing Kegel exercises correctly. Many people find it difficult to locate and engage their pelvic floor muscles, and may not be sure if they are performing Kegels correctly or effectively. With a biofeedback device, you can get immediate feedback on the activity of your pelvic floor muscles, which can help you to adjust your technique as needed.

In addition to providing feedback on your technique, biofeedback devices can also help you to track your progress over time. By measuring the strength and endurance of your pelvic floor muscles, you can see how your Kegel practice is improving over time. This can be particularly helpful for individuals who are using Kegel exercises to address specific health concerns, such as urinary incontinence or erectile dysfunction. Research has shown that biofeedback devices can be effective tools for improving pelvic floor muscle function in both men and women. A study published in the Journal of Urology found that biofeedback-assisted pelvic floor muscle exercises were more effective than standard exercises alone in improving symptoms of urinary incontinence in women. Similarly, a study published in the Journal of Sexual Medicine found that biofeedback-assisted pelvic floor muscle training was effective in improving erectile function in men with mild-to-moderate erectile dysfunction. It's important to note that while biofeedback devices can be useful tools, they are not necessary for successful Kegel practice. Many individuals are able to achieve significant improvements in pelvic floor muscle function with regular Kegel exercises alone. However, for individuals who are struggling to locate or engage their pelvic floor muscles, or who want to track their progress more closely, biofeedback devices can be a valuable addition to their Kegel practice. If you are considering using a biofeedback device to assist with your Kegel exercises, it's important to speak with a healthcare provider or pelvic floor therapist first.

They can help you to select an appropriate device and ensure that you are using it correctly and safely. Additionally, it's important to note that biofeedback devices can be expensive and may not be covered by insurance, so cost may be a consideration for some individuals. In summary, biofeedback devices can be useful tools for tracking your progress with Kegel exercises. They can provide real-time feedback on the activity of your pelvic floor muscles, help you to ensure that you are performing Kegels correctly, and allow you to track your progress over time. While not necessary for successful Kegel practice, biofeedback devices can be a valuable addition to your pelvic floor health routine.

## PARTNER EXERCISES FOR BETTER SEX AND INTIMACY

Partner exercises can be a fun and effective way to strengthen your pelvic floor muscles while also improving your sex life and overall intimacy. Not only do these exercises provide a unique opportunity to connect with your partner on a physical level, but they can also enhance your ability to experience pleasure during sex. Before diving into partner exercises, it's important to note that you should only engage in these activities with a willing and consenting partner. Additionally, if you or your partner have any medical conditions that affect your pelvic floor muscles, such as pelvic pain or urinary incontinence, it's important to consult with a healthcare professional before attempting any new exercises. One simple partner exercise is the "squeeze and release" technique. This exercise involves one partner lying on their back with their knees bent and feet flat on the ground, while the other partner kneels between their legs. The partner on the bottom then squeezes their pelvic floor muscles and holds for a few seconds before releasing. The partner on top can use their hands to provide resistance against the squeeze, making the exercise more challenging. Repeat for several sets, with each partner taking turns squeezing and resisting. Another partner exercise that can be effective is the "elevator" technique. Similar to the squeeze and release exercise, this technique involves one partner lying on their back with their knees bent and feet flat on the ground. The other partner kneels between their legs and uses their fingers to gently stimulate the pelvic area. The partner on the bottom then squeezes their pelvic floor muscles in a slow and controlled manner, imagining that they are lifting an elevator up to different floors. The partner on top can provide verbal cues to help guide the lift and release. Repeat for several sets, gradually increasing the number of "floors" lifted each time. For a more advanced partner exercise, try the "bridge and squeeze" technique. This exercise involves one partner lying on their back with their knees bent and feet flat on the ground, while the other partner stands at the end of the bed. The partner on the bottom then lifts their hips up into a bridge position, squeezing their pelvic floor muscles at the top of the lift. The partner standing at the end of the bed can provide resistance against the lift, making the exercise more challenging. Repeat for several sets, with each partner taking turns lifting and resisting. It's important to remember that partner exercises should always be done at a comfortable pace and intensity for both partners. It's also important to communicate openly with your partner throughout the exercise, checking in on comfort levels and providing feedback. In addition to strengthening your pelvic floor muscles, partner exercises can also have a positive impact on your overall sexual health and intimacy. By working together to improve your muscle tone and control, you may find that you are able to experience more intense orgasms, delay ejaculation or achieve longer-lasting erections, and increase your overall sexual confidence and satisfaction. In conclusion, partner exercises can be a fun and effective way to strengthen your pelvic floor muscles and enhance your sexual health and intimacy. By incorporating these exercises into your routine, you and your partner can improve your overall physical and emotional connection. Remember to always communicate openly with your partner and consult with a healthcare professional if you have any medical concerns.

# KEGELS FOR MEN

## BENEFITS OF KEGEL EXERCISES FOR MALE SEXUAL HEALTH

Kegel exercises are often associated with women's health, particularly during pregnancy and after childbirth. However, Kegels can also provide significant benefits for men's sexual health, particularly in the areas of erectile function and ejaculation control. Erectile dysfunction (ED) is a common condition that affects millions of men worldwide. ED can have a variety of causes, including underlying health conditions, psychological factors, and lifestyle factors. One of the key physiological factors in erectile function is blood flow to the penis. When the muscles in the pelvic floor are weak or damaged, blood flow can be impeded, leading to difficulty achieving and maintaining an erection. This is where Kegel exercises can help. By strengthening the muscles in the pelvic floor, men can improve blood flow to the penis and enhance their erectile function. Several studies have demonstrated a positive correlation between Kegel exercises and improved erectile function in men with mild to moderate ED. In one study published in the Journal of Sexual Medicine, men who performed Kegels for six months reported significant improvements in their ability to achieve and maintain erections, as well as increased sexual satisfaction.

Another sexual health benefit of Kegel exercises for men is improved ejaculation control. Premature ejaculation (PE) is a common sexual issue that can lead to frustration and embarrassment for both partners. PE is often caused by overactive pelvic floor muscles, which can trigger ejaculation prematurely. By performing Kegel exercises, men can learn to control their pelvic floor muscles more effectively and delay ejaculation as desired. In fact, Kegels are sometimes used as a treatment for PE, either on their own or in combination with other therapies. In a meta-analysis of multiple studies on Kegel exercises and PE published in Therapeutic Advances in Urology, researchers found that Kegels were effective in improving both subjective and objective measures of ejaculatory control. However, it's important to note that Kegels are not a one-size-fits-all solution for PE, and men with severe or persistent PE may need additional treatments or therapies. Aside from these specific sexual health benefits, Kegel exercises can also have more general health benefits for men. For example, strengthening the pelvic floor muscles can improve bladder and bowel control, which can be particularly important as men age and prostate health becomes a concern. Kegels may also help prevent or alleviate lower back pain, which can be a common issue for men who spend long hours sitting or standing. In summary, Kegel exercises are not just for women. Men can also benefit from regular Kegel practice, particularly in terms of improved erectile function and ejaculation control. By strengthening the muscles in the pelvic floor, men can improve their sexual health and overall quality of life. However, it's important to perform Kegels correctly and consistently to see the best results. If you're not sure how to do Kegels, or if you have any underlying health conditions that may affect your ability to do them safely, be sure to consult with your healthcare provider before starting a Kegel routine.

# HOW KEGELS CAN HELP WITH ERECTILE DYSFUNCTION, PREMATURE EJACULATION, AND PROSTATE HEALTH

For men, Kegel exercises can be a powerful tool for improving sexual function and overall health. Here are some of the ways that Kegels can specifically benefit men: Erectile Dysfunction: Erectile dysfunction (ED) is a common condition in which a man has difficulty achieving or maintaining an erection. Kegel exercises can help to strengthen the pelvic floor muscles, which play a key role in achieving and maintaining erections. By improving blood flow to the penis and increasing overall muscle tone, Kegels can help men with ED to achieve firmer, longer-lasting erections. One study found that after six months of regular Kegel practice, over 40% of men with ED saw significant improvement in their symptoms. Premature Ejaculation: Premature ejaculation (PE) is another common sexual problem that can be improved with Kegel exercises. By strengthening the pelvic floor muscles, men can gain greater control over their ejaculatory response, which can help to delay climax and improve sexual satisfaction for both partners. One study found that men who performed Kegel exercises for 12 weeks had a significant improvement in their ejaculatory control and sexual satisfaction. Prostate Health: The prostate gland is a small gland located between the bladder and the penis, and plays an important role in male sexual function and overall health. As men age, the prostate can become enlarged or inflamed, leading to urinary problems and other health issues. Regular Kegel practice can help to strengthen the pelvic floor muscles and improve blood flow to the prostate gland, reducing the risk of prostate problems and improving overall prostate health. In fact, studies have shown that men who regularly perform Kegels are less likely to develop prostate cancer. How to Do Kegels for

Men: Performing Kegel exercises is relatively simple, and can be done in the comfort of your own home. To perform a Kegel exercise, follow these steps: Find the right muscles: The first step is to locate the pelvic floor muscles. To do this, try to stop the flow of urine mid-stream. The muscles that you use to do this are your pelvic floor muscles. Practice the exercise: Once you have located the pelvic floor muscles, you can begin practicing the Kegel exercise. Squeeze the muscles tight and hold for 5-10 seconds, then release and relax for the same amount of time. Repeat this cycle of squeezing and releasing 10-15 times in a row, several times per day. Add resistance: To make your Kegel exercises more challenging and effective, you can add resistance by using a Kegel exerciser or a weighted cone. These devices can help to strengthen the pelvic floor muscles more quickly and effectively than standard Kegel exercises. Kegel exercises can be a highly effective tool for improving sexual function and overall health for men. By strengthening the pelvic floor muscles, men can improve their erections, control their ejaculatory response, and reduce the risk of prostate problems. If you're experiencing any of these issues, consider adding Kegel exercises to your daily routine to see if they can help. As always, it's important to consult with a healthcare professional before beginning any new exercise routine.

## SPECIFIC EXERCISES FOR MEN, INCLUDING REVERSE KEGELS AND PELVIC FLOOR STRETCHES

Kegel exercises are not just for women. Men can also benefit greatly from strengthening their pelvic floor muscles, which can improve their sexual health, urinary continence, and even prostate health. In this chapter, we will discuss specific exercises that men can do to strengthen their pelvic floor muscles, including reverse Kegels and pelvic floor stretches. Reverse Kegels Kegels are typically associated with squeezing or contracting the pelvic floor muscles, but the opposite motion – releasing or relaxing those muscles – is also important. Reverse Kegels involve consciously relaxing and lengthening the pelvic floor muscles. This can help counteract the effects of chronic tension in the pelvic floor, which can contribute to urinary and sexual problems. To perform a reverse Kegel, follow these steps: Sit or lie down in a comfortable position and take a few deep breaths to relax. Focus your attention on the muscles between your scrotum and anus (the perineum). Imagine that you are trying to stretch and lengthen those muscles, as if you were trying to push something out of your body. Keep your abdominal muscles relaxed and avoid tensing your buttocks or thighs. Hold the stretch for a few seconds, then release and relax for a few seconds before repeating. Pelvic Floor Stretches Stretching is an important part of any exercise routine, and the pelvic floor muscles are no exception. Tight or tense pelvic floor muscles can contribute to pain, discomfort, and dysfunction, so regular stretching can help maintain flexibility and mobility. Here are two effective pelvic floor stretches that men can try: Happy Baby Pose Lie on your back with your knees bent and feet flat on the floor. Bring your knees up toward your chest, then reach down and grab the outsides of your feet with your hands. Use your arms to gently pull your knees down toward your armpits, keeping your feet flexed. Hold the stretch for 30 seconds to 1 minute, breathing deeply. Butterfly Pose Sit on the floor with your knees bent and the soles of your feet touching. Gently press your elbows into your inner thighs and use your hands to push your knees down toward the floor. Hold the stretch for 30 seconds to 1 minute, breathing deeply. Incorporating Kegels into Your Routine While these specific exercises can be helpful, it's important to remember that Kegel exercises are just one part of a comprehensive pelvic floor strengthening routine. Men can also benefit from incorporating Kegels into their overall fitness routine, such as by doing Kegels during strength training or cardio workouts. In addition, lifestyle factors such as diet, hydration, and stress management can all affect pelvic floor health, so addressing these factors can help optimize the benefits of Kegel exercises. In conclusion, men can benefit greatly from regular pelvic floor exercises, including Kegels, reverse Kegels, and pelvic floor stretches. By incorporating these exercises into their routine and addressing other factors that can affect pelvic floor health, men can improve their sexual function, urinary continence, and overall quality of life.

Where can I do these exercises?

When you first start doing the exercises, find a place where you can do them without being interrupted. After you have done them for a while, you can practice the exercises anytime and anywhere (e.g. watching TV, standing in line, driving a car, etc.)

Note: It often takes 6 to 12 weeks to see results, if you do these exercises regularly.

Things you can do to help your pelvic floor muscles:

After a surgery, always squeeze your pelvic floor muscles when you:

• Sit up from lying down

• Stand up from a sitting position

• Lift something heavy

Remember to:

• Keep breathing while doing the exercises

• Only squeeze and lift

• Do NOT tighten your buttocks

• Keep your thighs relaxed

• Don't strain when using your bowels

• Eat fruit and vegetables

• Drink 6 to 8 glasses of water daily

• Keep your weight within the right range for your height and age


How long and how many?

When you are first starting out, it is common to find that you can only hold a Kegel for 3-6 seconds, and that performing 3-6 repetitions causes muscle fatigue. When this happens, you are usually performing the exercise correctly. If you find you can hold it for much longer right away, recheck your technique. For patients with incontinence or pelvic floor weakness, it is important to concentrate on correctly performing the technique and gradually improving the muscle quality and tone, even though you may be weak first starting out.

## Advanced Kegel Exercises

1. Prolonged Contractions:

Step 1: Begin by emptying your bladder to ensure comfort during the exercise.

Step 2: Sit or lie down in a comfortable position.

Step 3: Identify your pelvic floor muscles by tightening them as if you were trying to stop the flow of urine or prevent gas release.

Step 4: Once you've isolated the muscles, contract them and hold for an extended period (e.g., 10 seconds or more).

Step 5: Release the contraction slowly and completely.

Step 6: Rest for a few seconds between contractions.

Step 7: Repeat the prolonged contractions for a set number of repetitions, gradually increasing the duration as your strength improves.

Note: Focus on maintaining a smooth and controlled contraction throughout the exercise. It's crucial to avoid holding your breath or tensing other muscles in your body.

2. Incorporating Resistance (e.g., Kegel Balls):

Step 1: Choose appropriate Kegel balls or resistance devices designed for pelvic floor exercises.

Step 2: Clean the device thoroughly according to the manufacturer's instructions.

Step 3: Apply a water-based lubricant to the device to ease insertion.

Step 4: Relax your body and insert the Kegel balls or device into your rectum or vagina, depending on the design.

Step 5: Identify your pelvic floor muscles and contract them around the inserted device.

Step 6: Hold the contraction for a few seconds, then release.

Step 7:Perform a series of contractions and releases, gradually increasing the duration and intensity.

Step 8: Remove the device carefully after completing the exercise.

3. Elevator Contractions:

• Step 1: Gradually tighten your pelvic floor muscles as if you are going up an elevator.

• Step 2: Start with a gentle contraction and progressively increase the intensity, as if stopping at different floors.

• Step 3: Hold the highest contraction for a few seconds, then release in a controlled manner, gradually descending.

4. Quick Contractions:

• Step 1: Contract and release your pelvic floor muscles rapidly in quick succession.

• Step 2: Focus on the speed of the contractions while maintaining control.

• Step 3: Perform these quick contractions for a set duration or number of repetitions.

5. Side-to-Side Contractions:

• Step 1: Contract your pelvic floor muscles while also engaging the muscles on the sides of your pelvic area.

• Step 2: Hold the contraction, feeling the engagement along the sides.

• Step 3: Release the contraction and repeat, ensuring equal engagement on both sides.

6. Flutter Kicks:

• Step 1: Rapidly alternate between contracting and releasing your pelvic floor muscles, creating a fluttering sensation.

• Step 2: Maintain a steady rhythm throughout the exercise.

• Step 3: Gradually increase the speed as you become more comfortable with the movement.

7. Bridge Pose with Kegels:

• Step 1: Lie on your back with knees bent and feet flat on the floor.

• Step 2: Lift your hips off the ground into a bridge pose.

• Step 3: While holding the bridge, perform Kegel contractions, focusing on the engagement in the pelvic area.

• Step 4: Lower your hips back down and repeat the sequence.

8. Squats with Kegels:

• Step 1: Perform a squat by lowering your body as if sitting back into a chair.

• Step 2: As you rise back up, contract your pelvic floor muscles.

• Step 3: Repeat the squatting motion while incorporating Kegel contractions.

9. Resistance Band Kegels:

• Step 1: Attach a resistance band around your thighs, just above the knees.

• Step 2: Perform Kegel contractions against the resistance of the band.

• Step 3: Focus on maintaining proper form and control throughout the exercise.

10. Balloon Breathing with Kegels:

• Step 1: Inhale deeply, expanding your diaphragm and pelvic floor.

• Step 2: Contract your pelvic floor muscles as you exhale, imagining you're blowing up a balloon.

• Step 3: Inhale again, allowing the pelvic floor to relax. Repeat the cycle.

Note: Consult with a healthcare professional before using any resistance devices, especially if you have pelvic health concerns. Ensure the device is appropriate for your individual needs and follow any specific instructions provided by the manufacturer.

Remember to start gradually with advanced Kegel exercises and listen to your body. If you experience any pain or discomfort, it's advisable to consult with a healthcare provider before continuing.

Do your Kegel exercises well.

Fewer good squeezes are better than a lot of half-hearted ones.

If you are not sure that you are doing the squeezes right, or if you do not see a change in symptoms after 3 months, contact your doctor's office asking how to for help.

## 11. Isometric Contractions:

• Step 1: Sit or stand comfortably.

• Step 2: Contract your pelvic floor muscles without moving any other part of your body.

• Step 3: Hold the contraction for an extended period, gradually increasing the duration over time.

• Step 4: Release the contraction slowly and completely.

12. Dynamic Kegels with Leg Lifts:

• Step 1: Lie on your back with legs extended.

• Step 2: Lift one leg at a time while simultaneously contracting your pelvic floor muscles.

• Step 3: Lower the leg and switch to the other side.

• Step 4: Repeat the leg lifts, coordinating with Kegel contractions.

13. Pelvic Clock Exercise:

• Step 1: Visualize a clock over your pelvic area.

• Step 2: Contract your pelvic floor muscles at 12 o'clock, then relax.

• Step 3: Move to 3 o'clock, contract, and relax. Repeat for 6 o'clock and 9 o'clock.

• Step 4: Continue the clock-wise pattern, engaging different areas of the pelvic floor.

14. Pilates Ball Squeezes:

• Step 1: Sit on a Pilates ball with feet flat on the floor.

• Step 2: Squeeze the ball between your thighs while simultaneously contracting your pelvic floor.

• Step 3: Release the squeeze and the pelvic floor contraction.

• Step 4: Repeat the exercise, focusing on control and coordination.

15. Deep Squats with Kegels:

• Step 1: Perform a deep squat, lowering your body as far as comfortable.

• Step 2: Contract your pelvic floor muscles at the lowest point of the squat.

• Step 3: Rise back up, releasing the pelvic floor contraction.

• Step 4: Repeat, ensuring proper squat form and pelvic floor engagement.

16. Breath-Linked Kegels:

• Step 1: Inhale deeply, expanding your diaphragm.

• Step 2: As you exhale, contract your pelvic floor muscles.

• Step 3: Inhale again, releasing the pelvic floor contraction.

• Step 4: Coordinate Kegels with your breath, focusing on smooth transitions.

17. Seated Butterfly Kegels:

• Step 1: Sit with your back straight and the soles of your feet together.

• Step 2: Allow your knees to fall to the sides, creating a butterfly shape.

• Step 3: Contract and release your pelvic floor muscles while maintaining the butterfly position.

18. Plank with Pelvic Tilt:

• Step 1: Assume a plank position with your body in a straight line.

• Step 2: Tilt your pelvis upward, engaging your pelvic floor muscles.

• Step 3: Return to a neutral plank position, releasing the pelvic floor contraction.

• Step 4: Repeat the pelvic tilt, focusing on core stability.

19. Kegel Marching:

• Step 1: Lie on your back with knees bent.

• Step 2: Lift one leg at a time while contracting your pelvic floor muscles.

• Step 3: Alternate legs in a marching motion, coordinating with Kegel contractions.

20. Kegel and Abdominal Co-activation:

• Step 1: Sit or stand with good posture.

• Step 2: Contract your pelvic floor muscles while simultaneously engaging your abdominal muscles.

• Step 3: Hold the co-contraction for a few seconds, then release.

• Step 4: Repeat, focusing on the synergy between pelvic floor and abdominal engagement.

## Establishing a Routine

### The Frequency And Duration Of Kegel Exercises

The frequency and duration of Kegel exercises can vary depending on individual needs, goals, and any specific recommendations from healthcare professionals. However, here are general guidelines that can serve as a starting point:

- Frequency:
- Beginners: Start with a routine of 3 sets of 10 repetitions per day.
- Intermediate: Gradually increase to 4 sets of 15-20 repetitions per day.
- Advanced: Aim for 5 sets of 20-30 repetitions per day.
- Duration:
- Contraction Time: Initially, hold each contraction for about 3-5 seconds.
- Rest Time: Allow 3-5 seconds of rest between contractions.
- Progression: Over time, gradually increase the duration of contractions to 10 seconds

or more, and extend the rest period as needed.

- Consistency:
- Daily Routine: Perform Kegel exercises daily for optimal results.
- Incorporate Into Routine: Consider integrating Kegels into your daily activities, such as during moments of routine, like brushing your teeth or waiting at a traffic light.
- Monitoring Progress:
- Keep a Journal: Maintain a Kegel exercise journal to track your progress, including the number of sets, repetitions, and any changes in symptoms or benefits.
- Reassess Regularly: Periodically reassess your routine and make adjustments based on improvements or changes in your pelvic health.
- Special Considerations:
- Postpartum Women: Women who have recently given birth may start with gentler exercises and gradually progress as recommended by their healthcare provider.
- Individual Needs: Adjust the frequency and duration based on your individual comfort

level, response to the exercises, and any guidance from healthcare professionals.

Remember that consistency is key, and it may take several weeks to months to notice significant improvements. If you experience any discomfort or have specific concerns, it's advisable to consult with a healthcare provider, particularly if you have a history of pelvic floor issues, recent surgery, or other medical conditions. Additionally, healthcare professionals may provide personalized recommendations based on your specific situation and goals.

## Incorporating Kegel Exercises Into Your Daily Activities

Here are some creative ways to integrate Kegels into your day:

- Morning Routine:
- Perform Kegels while brushing your teeth or during your morning skincare routine.
- Incorporate Kegels into your stretching or yoga routine.
- Commute or Driving:
- Do Kegels while sitting in traffic or waiting at a stoplight.
- Alternate short and long contractions to keep things interesting.
- Desk Exercises:
- Sit on a stability ball instead of a chair to engage your core and pelvic floor muscles.
- Incorporate discreet Kegels during meetings or while working at your desk.
- TV Time:
- Perform Kegels during commercial breaks or while watching TV.
- Use the duration of your favorite show as a timer for sets of Kegel exercises.

- Phone Use:
- Link Kegels to phone activities, such as texting or scrolling through social media.
- Create a habit of doing Kegels every time you answer a phone call.
- Mealtime:
- Perform Kegels while waiting for your food to heat in the microwave.
- Use the time it takes to chew your food as a cue for Kegel exercises.
- Before and After Bathroom Breaks:
- Perform a set of Kegels before and after using the restroom.
- Use this routine as a reminder to stay consistent with your exercises.
- Bedtime Routine:
- Incorporate Kegels into your nighttime routine, such as while washing your face or getting ready for bed.
- Wind down with a few minutes of relaxation and deep breathing, incorporating Kegels.
- Exercising:
- Integrate Kegels into your regular workout routine, especially during strength training exercises.

- Combine Kegels with cardiovascular activities like walking or jogging.
- Mindful Moments:
- Practice mindfulness and perform Kegels during moments of reflection or meditation.
- Use cues from your surroundings, such as the sound of a bell, to prompt a set of Kegel exercises.

Remember to focus on proper technique during these activities and adjust the intensity based on your comfort level. Consistency is key, so finding natural cues in your daily routine can help you establish a regular Kegel exercise habit. If you have specific concerns or conditions, it's always advisable to consult with a healthcare professional for personalized guidance.

## Conclusion

Do not perform the exercises too much.

Do not do more than 100 Kegel's in one day, as this can tire out the muscles and make you leak more. Start slow and gradually increase the amount of exercise.

Remember to breathe during the exercises. Holding your breath may put extra pressure on your pelvic muscles.

www.ingramcontent.com/pod-product-compliance
Lightning Source LLC
Chambersburg PA
CBHW070959290526
45795CB00005B/1700